Nutrition in Every Bite: A Collection of Kitchen Health Marvels"

Content

Introduction to Nutrient-Rich Eating

In this opening chapter, readers embark on a journey into the fundamental principles of nutrient-rich eating, laying the foundation for a healthy and balanced lifestyle. The chapter covers:

1. **The Essence of Nutrient-Rich Foods:** Explore the concept of nutrient density and understand how it forms the cornerstone of a health-focused diet.

2. **Building Blocks of Nutrition:** Introduce readers to the essential macronutrients (carbohydrates, proteins, and fats) and micronutrients (vitamins and minerals) that contribute to overall well-being.

3. **The Role of Whole Foods:** Emphasize the importance of incorporating whole, unprocessed foods into daily meals and the benefits they bring to the body.

4. **Balancing Act**: Discuss the significance of striking a balance between different nutrients, avoiding extremes, and customizing diets to individual needs.

5. **The Impact of Nutrition on Health**:   Delve into the profound effects of a nutrient-rich diet on physical health, mental well-being, and longevity.

6. **Myth-busting Nutritional Misconceptions**: Address common misconceptions about diet and nutrition, fostering a clearer understanding of what constitutes a healthy eating plan.

7. **Practical Tips for Nutrient-Rich Living**: Provide actionable tips for integrating nutrient-rich foods into everyday meals, making it accessible for readers to start their journey towards a healthier lifestyle.

By the end of this chapter, readers will have a solid grasp of the importance of nutrient-rich eating, setting the stage for the exploration of specific foods, recipes, and dietary practices in the subsequent chapters of "Nutrition in Every Bite.

Power of Superfoods: Incorporating Them Into Daily Meals

The world of superfoods, exploring their nutritional prowess and learning how to seamlessly integrate these nutritional powerhouses into everyday meals. The chapter unfolds as follows:

1. **Understanding Superfoods**: Provide an in-depth overview of what qualifies as a superfood, highlighting nutrient density, antioxidants, and other health-promoting properties.

2. **Superfood Spotlight:** Showcase a selection of diverse superfoods, ranging from well-known ones like kale, blueberries, and quinoa to lesser-known gems such as spirulina, chia seeds, and moringa.

3. **Nutrient Profiles:** Break down the nutritional content of featured superfoods, elucidating the specific vitamins, minerals, and other beneficial compounds they offer.

4. **Health Benefits:** Explore the myriad health benefits associated with regular consumption of superfoods, including improved immune function, enhanced cognitive health, and increased energy levels.

5. **Practical Tips for Incorporation:** Provide practical and creative ways to incorporate superfoods into daily meals, ensuring that readers can easily integrate these nutritional powerhouses into their existing diets.

6. **Superfood Recipes:** Include a selection of easy-to-follow recipes that showcase the versatility of superfoods, demonstrating how they can be used in smoothies, salads, main dishes, and snacks.

7. **Navigating the Market:** Offer guidance on sourcing high-quality superfoods, whether fresh, frozen, or in powder form, and share tips on budget-friendly options.

By the end of this chapter, readers will have gained a comprehensive understanding of superfoods, equipped with the knowledge and inspiration to elevate their daily meals with nutrient-rich additions. This sets the stage for further exploration of holistic and health-conscious eating in subsequent chapters.

Essential Nutrients Demystified: A Guide to Vitamins and Minerals

This chapter provides readers with a thorough exploration of essential nutrients, unraveling the complexities of vitamins and minerals. It serves as a foundational guide to understanding the crucial role these elements play in maintaining optimal health. The chapter unfolds as follows:

1. **Vitamins**: The Alphabet of Wellness Break down the various vitamins, from A to K, outlining their functions, sources, and the specific health benefits associated with each.

2. **Minerals:** The Building Blocks of Vitality Explore essential minerals such as calcium, magnesium, iron, and zinc, elucidating their roles in bodily functions and the consequences of deficiencies.

3. **Synergy and Interactions:** Discuss how vitamins and minerals often work synergistically, emphasizing the importance of a well-rounded and varied diet to ensure comprehensive nutrient intake.

4. **Daily Requirements:** Provide recommended daily allowances for vitamins and minerals, helping readers understand the quantities needed for optimal health and where to find them in food sources.

5. **Nutrient Absorption** Delve into factors affecting nutrient absorption, such as bioavailability and the influence of dietary choices, to empower readers to maximize the benefits of the nutrients they consume.

6. **Balancing Act:** Avoiding Excess and Deficiency Address the risks associated with both nutrient excess and deficiency, offering practical tips for achieving a balanced intake through dietary choices.

7. **Supplementation Considerations** Discuss the role of supplements in filling potential nutritional gaps, highlighting instances where supplementation may be beneficial and when it's preferable to rely on whole food sources.

By the end of this chapter, readers will have gained a comprehensive understanding of the essential vitamins and minerals vital for their well-being. Armed with this knowledge, they'll be better equipped to make informed dietary choices that support optimal health and vitality.

Hydration Heroes: Infused Waters and Herbal Teas

This chapter immerses readers in the world of hydrating and health-boosting beverages, focusing on infused waters and herbal teas. It explores the art of crafting refreshing drinks that not only quench thirst but also contribute to overall well-being. The chapter unfolds as follows:

1. **The Foundation of Hydration:** Understanding Water Emphasize the importance of proper hydration for bodily functions, highlighting the role of water in digestion, metabolism, and overall cellular health.

2. **Infused Waters:** Nature's Flavored Elixirs- Showcase a variety of infused water recipes using fruits, herbs, and spices, offering both delightful flavors and added nutritional benefits.

3. **Herbal Teas:** Sipping Wellness- Introduce the world of herbal teas, exploring the health benefits associated with different herbs and their potential to address common ailments.

4. **Tea Varieties and Their Properties**: Delve into the diverse range of herbal teas, such as chamomile for

relaxation, peppermint for digestion, and hibiscus for antioxidants, providing a comprehensive guide to their properties.

5. **DIY Infusions:** Crafting Your Hydration Experience
 - Empower readers to experiment with creating their own infused waters and herbal tea blends, fostering creativity in the kitchen.

6. **Beyond Hydration:** Functional Infusions- Explore functional infusions that go beyond mere hydration, incorporating ingredients known for their specific health benefits, such as turmeric for anti-inflammatory effects or ginger for digestive support.

7. **Choosing Quality Ingredients**: Offer guidance on selecting fresh, high-quality ingredients for infusions and teas, whether from the garden, local markets, or specialty stores.

By the end of this chapter, readers will have discovered a new dimension to hydration, transforming it from a mundane necessity into a flavorful and health-enhancing experience. This knowledge equips them with tools to stay hydrated while indulging in the rich, diverse world of infused waters and herbal teas.

Plant-Based Wonders: Elevating Your Diet with Vegetarian Delights

This chapter invites readers to explore the vibrant world of plant-based eating, emphasizing the nutritional richness and culinary diversity of vegetarian dishes. It serves as a guide to incorporating more plant-based wonders into daily meals. The chapter unfolds as follows:

1. **The Essence of Plant-Based Eating:** Introduce the concept of plant-based eating, emphasizing the focus on whole, plant-derived foods and the associated health benefits.

2. **Nutrient-Rich Vegetarian Staples:** Showcase a variety of nutrient-dense vegetarian staples, including legumes whole grains, nuts, seeds, and a colorful array of fruits and vegetables.

3. **Protein Power:** Plant-Based Sources- Explore plant-based protein sources, debunking myths about protein deficiency in vegetarian diets and highlighting the protein-rich potential of beans, lentils, tofu, and more.

4. **Essential Nutrients in Plant Foods**: Break down the essential vitamins, minerals, and other beneficial compounds found in plant-based foods, illustrating how a well-rounded plant-based diet can provide a spectrum of nutrients.

5. **Flavorful Meat Alternatives**: Introduce delicious meat alternatives such as tempeh, seitan, and jack - fruit , showcasing their versatility in creating satisfying and nutritionally dense meals.

6. **Balancing Macronutrients in Plant-Based Meals**: Provide guidance on achieving a balanced macronutrient profile in plant-based meals, ensuring readers meet their energy and nutritional needs.

7. **Global Vegetarian Cuisine:** A Culinary Journey- Explore diverse vegetarian cuisines from around the world, offering readers a taste of flavorful and culturally rich plant-based dishes.

8. **Practical Tips for Transitioning:** Offer practical advice and tips for those interested in transitioning to a more plant-based diet, making the shift accessible and enjoyable.

By the end of this chapter, readers will have gained insights into the nutritional bounty of plant-based eating, empowering them to embrace a more diverse and health-conscious culinary lifestyle. This sets the stage for further exploration of vegetarian recipes and culinary adventures in subsequent chapters.

Protein-packed Pleasures: A Balanced Approach to Meat and Alternatives

In this chapter, readers embark on a comprehensive exploration of protein-rich foods, striking a balance between animal-derived sources and plant-based alternatives. The focus is on fostering a well-rounded, protein-packed diet that supports overall health. The chapter unfolds as follows:

1. **Understanding the Importance of Protein:** Establish the fundamental role of protein in bodily functions, including muscle repair, immune support, and the synthesis of essential molecules.

2. **Animal-Based Protein Sources:** Explore a variety of animal-based protein sources, such as lean meats, poultry, fish, and dairy products, emphasizing the nutritional value they bring to the table.

3. **Navigating Healthy Fats in Animal Proteins:** Discuss the importance of choosing lean cuts and incorporating sources of healthy fats from animal proteins, such as omega-3 fatty acids from fish.

4. **Plant-Based Protein Alternatives** Showcase a diverse

range of plant-based protein alternatives, including legumes, tofu, tempeh, quinoa, and edamame, illustrating their protein content and versatility.

5. **Combining Proteins for Optimal Nutrition:** Provide insights into protein combining, exploring how to create complementary protein pairs for a more comprehensive amino acid profile in both plant and animal-based meals.

6. **Protein and Physical Activity**: Discuss the correlation between protein intake and physical activity, offering guidance on protein needs for individuals engaged in different levels of exercise and fitness.

7. **Protein for Special Diets** Address specific dietary considerations, such as protein requirements for vegetarians, vegans, and individuals with dietary restrictions or allergies.

8. **Protein-Rich Recipes**: Include a selection of protein-rich recipes that showcase the delicious possibilities of incorporating both animal and plant-based protein sources into everyday meals.

By the end of this chapter, readers will have gained a holistic understanding of protein as a crucial component of a balanced diet. Armed with knowledge about diverse protein sources, they'll be able to craft meals that not only satisfy taste buds but also provide essential nutrients for overall well-being. This knowledge serves as a valuable resource as readers continue their journey toward a protein-packed and nutritionally balanced lifestyle.

Healthy Fats: Navigating the World of Good Fats and Their Benefits

This chapter guides readers through the intricate landscape of dietary fats, highlighting the importance of healthy fats in maintaining overall well-being. It explores the diverse world of fats, dispelling misconceptions and offering practical insights for making informed dietary choices. The chapter unfolds as follows:

1. **The Role of Fats in the Body**: Establish the vital functions of fats, including energy storage, hormone production, and the absorption of fat-soluble vitamins (A, D, E, K).

2. **Understanding Healthy Fats vs. Unhealthy Fats**: Differentiate between healthy fats (monounsaturated and polyunsaturated fats) and unhealthy fats (saturated and trans fats), explaining their respective effects on heart health and overall wellness.

3. **Omega-3 Fatty Acids:** The Heart-Healthy Essential - Spotlight the benefits of omega-3 fatty acids, found in fatty fish, flaxseeds, chia seeds, and walnuts, and their

positive impact on cardiovascular health and inflammation.

4. **Sources of Healthy Fats**: Provide an extensive list of foods rich in healthy fats, encompassing avocados, olive oil, nuts, seeds, and fatty fish, empowering readers to diversify their fat intake.

5. **Balancing Fat Intake in the Diet**: Offer practical guidelines on achieving a balanced fat intake, emphasizing portion control and the importance of variety in fat sources.

6. **Cooking with Healthy Fats:** Explore optimal cooking methods for preserving the nutritional integrity of healthy fats, as well as the smoke points of different oils.

7. **Fats and Brain Health**: Discuss the role of fats in cognitive function and brain health, shedding light on the connection between dietary fats and mental well-being.

8. **Myths and Facts about Fats**: Address common myths surrounding dietary fats, such as the misconception that all fats contribute to weight gain, providing evidence-based information to dispel misinformation.

By the end of this chapter, readers will have gained a nuanced understanding of the significance of healthy fats in a balanced diet. Armed with practical knowledge, they'll be equipped to make conscious and informed choices to optimize their fat intake for improved overall health.

Mindful Eating Practices: Bringing Awareness to Every Bite

This chapter delves into the concept of mindful eating, exploring the profound impact of cultivating awareness during meals. It provides readers with practical insights and techniques to foster a mindful approach to eating, promoting not only physical health but also a deeper connection with food. The chapter unfolds as follows:

1. **The Art of Mindful Eating**: Introduce the fundamental principles of mindful eating, emphasizing the importance of being fully present and engaged during meals.

2. **Mind-Body Connection:** Understanding Hunger and Satisfaction- Explore the mind-body connection in relation to hunger and satisfaction, guiding readers to recognize and respond to genuine hunger cues.

3. **Savoring Flavors:** Enhancing the Dining Experience
   - Encourage readers to savor the flavors, textures, and aromas of their meals, transforming eating into a sensory experience that goes beyond mere sustenance.

4. **Breaking Free from Emotional Eating**
   - Address the connection between emotions and

eating habits, providing strategies to break free from emotional triggers and establish a healthier relationship with food.

5. **Portion Awareness:** Finding Balance in Serving Sizes- Offer practical tips for portion control, helping readers develop an intuitive sense of appropriate serving sizes to support overall health.

6. **Chewing and Digestion:** The Importance of Slow and Steady- Illuminate the benefits of chewing food thoroughly, not only for digestion but also for the enjoyment of each bite and the promotion of a mindful eating experience.

7. **Creating a Nourishing Environment**
   - Discuss the impact of the dining environment on mindful eating, from minimizing distractions to cultivating a positive and peaceful atmosphere.

8. **Mindful Eating Practices in Everyday Life**
   - Provide actionable steps for incorporating mindful eating practices into daily life, whether at home, work, or social gatherings.

9. **Mindful Eating and Weight Management**
   - Explore the connection between mindful eating and sustainable weight management, highlighting the potential benefits of a mindful approach in making healthier food choices.

By the end of this chapter, readers will have gained a deeper understanding of the transformative power of mindful eating. Armed with practical tools and techniques, they'll be empowered to approach meals with heightened awareness, fostering a more intentional and enjoyable relationship with food. This chapter serves as a valuable resource for individuals seeking to cultivate mindful eating practices as a cornerstone of their overall well-being.

Colorful Plates: The Importance of a Diverse Diet

This chapter celebrates the vibrant tapestry of nutrition found in a diverse and colorful diet. It explores the significance of consuming a wide array of fruits, vegetables, and other food groups, highlighting the nutritional benefits and promoting overall health. The chapter unfolds as follows:

1. **The Nutritional Spectrum of Colors**
   - Introduce the concept that the colors of foods represent different nutrients and antioxidants, emphasizing the importance of creating visually diverse meals.

2. **Phytonutrients and Antioxidants:** The Power of Plant Pigments- Explore the role of phytonutrients and anti-oxidants in plant pigments, discussing their potential health benefits and protective properties against oxidative stress.

3. **Eating the Rainbow:** A Guide to Colorful Nutrition
   - Guide readers through the rainbow of fruits and vegetables, showcasing the unique nutritional profiles of different colors and encouraging a varied and balanced diet.

4. **Beyond Fruits and Veggies:** Diversifying Food Groups
- Expand the concept of diversity to include a variety of food groups, incorporating whole grains, lean proteins, and healthy fats for a comprehensive nutritional approach.

5. **Gut Health and Diversity**
   - Discuss the connection between a diverse diet and gut health, exploring how different foods promote a flourishing microbiome and contribute to overall digestive well-being.

6. **Reducing Nutrient Gaps Through Diversity**
   - Address the risk of nutrient deficiencies associated with a limited diet, emphasizing how a diverse range of foods helps fill nutritional gaps and ensures comprehensive nutrient intake.

7. **Adventurous Eating:** Exploring New Flavors and Cuisines- Encourage readers to step outside their culinary comfort zones, trying new ingredients, flavors, and recipes to enhance the diversity of their meals.

8. **Practical Tips for Achieving Dietary Diversity**
   - Provide actionable tips for incorporating a variety of foods into daily meals, including meal planning, exploring local markets, and experimenting with different cooking methods.

By the end of this chapter, readers will have gained a profound appreciation for the nutritional benefits of a diverse and colorful diet. Empowered with practical insights and inspiration, they'll be motivated to create visually appealing, nutritionally rich meals that contribute to their overall well-being. This chapter serves as a valuable resource for individuals seeking to enhance their dietary diversity and embrace the spectrum of flavors and nutrients found in a vibrant and varied eating pattern.

Guilt-Free Indulgences: Desserts That Nourish Body and Soul

This chapter invites readers into the realm of guilt-free indulgences the art of creating desserts that not only satisfy sweet cravings but also contribute to overall well-being. It aims to redefine the perception of desserts by emphasizing nourishing ingredients and mindful consumption. The chapter unfolds as follows:

1. **The Psychology of Desserts:** Balancing Pleasure and Wellness- Explore the emotional and psychological aspects of dessert consumption, discussing the importance of balancing the enjoyment of treats with overall well-being.

2. **Nourishing Sweeteners:** Beyond Refined Sugar
   - Introduce alternative sweeteners such as honey, maple syrup, and dates, discussing their nutritional benefits and how they can be incorporated into healthier dessert recipes.

3. **Whole Ingredients:** Elevating Desserts with Nutrient-Rich Elements- Emphasize the use of whole, minimally processed ingredients in dessert recipes, such as whole grains, nuts, seeds, and fruits, to enhance the nutritional content.

4. **Mindful Portions:** Savoring Sweet Moments- Discuss the concept of mindful indulgence, encouraging readers to savor smaller portions of desserts while fully enjoying the flavors and textures.

5. **Reducing Processed Additives:** Creating Clean Treats
   - Highlight the drawbacks of processed additives in traditional desserts and provide alternatives to create cleaner, more wholesome treats.

6. **Balancing Indulgence with Nutritional Value**
   - Showcase recipes that strike a balance between indulgence and nutritional value, incorporating ingredients with health benefits, such as antioxidants, fiber, and essential nutrients.

7. **Celebrating Seasonal Flavors: Freshness in Every Bite**
   - Explore the use of seasonal fruits and flavors in desserts, emphasizing the connection between desserts and the natural rhythm of produce availability.

8. **Homemade Goodness: Crafting Desserts from Scratch**
   - Encourage readers to embrace homemade desserts, empowering them to control ingredients, experiment with flavors, and infuse love into their culinary creations.

9. **Family-Friendly Treats:** Nourishing Bonds Through Desserts- Discuss the role of desserts in family traditions, providing family-friendly recipes that bring joy and nourishment to shared moments.

10. **Desserts for Special Occasions:** Elevating the Celebration- Explore the art of creating special occasion desserts that contribute to the joy of celebrations while maintaining a focus on mindful and nourishing ingredients.

By the end of this chapter, readers will have gained a newfound appreciation for desserts that not only satisfy the sweet tooth but also contribute to their overall well-being. Armed with a collection of guilt-free indulgence recipes, they'll be inspired to enjoy sweet treats mindfully, embracing the pleasure of desserts without compromising their commitment to a health-conscious lifestyle. This chapter serves as a delightful conclusion to the journey of creating a balanced and nourishing approach to eating.